I Weight No More

The Ultimate Motivational Weight Loss Plan

The road to victory is here

To stay fit for life
To feel good about you
To find exceptional skills
To be the leader of your destiny

I Weight No More

Your Weight is Over

Mera Lord

Writers Club Press
San Jose New York Lincoln Shanghai

I Weight No More
Your Weight is Over

Writers Club Press
an imprint of iUniverse.com, Inc.

For information address:
iUniverse.com, Inc.
5220 S 16th, Ste. 200
Lincoln, NE 68512
www.iuniverse.com

ISBN: 0-595-20178-4

Printed in the United States of America

To my husband, Bob, whose honesty and sense of humor made my life as light as a feather, who led me to believe in no boundaries, to stay focused, and to go after my dreams. To my children, Nina and Sebastian, who connected Heaven and Earth to me.

EPIGRAPH

I have written this book for you the reader,
To be able to find your own green thumb,
To nurture your roots,
And to be able to blossom.

CONTENTS

FOREWORD

I have written this book because I feel the tremendous need and a sense of hopelessness that most people have toward achieving their ideal weight.

I like to mention that I have been through the pain. The pain of walking my days in the shadow of uncertainty. The shadow of not living fully.

My mission is to show you how simple and easy it is to achieve your ideal weight and stay fit for life. To be the best you can be and enjoy the life to it's fullest.

I have concentrated only on the very basic rules and yet the most important ones that makes a big difference in the long run.

This book is focused on learning the skills you need for staying fit for life. A workbook to guide you in managing your diet and fitness easily.

The simple methods in this book will show you step by step how to become fit. It doesn't matter how old or how over weight you are, you will be able to achieve your goal. The important thing is following the rules and being consistence.

This book will show you how easy it is to reach your goals.

This is a motivational weight loss plan concentrating on solutions rather than dieting alone.

It is true that we are creatures of habits, but when we know where the wrong habits are, only then we can undo the wrong by learning the right skills.

Keep this in mind; consistently work toward achieving your goal.

And here is the plan.

The Ultimate Goal

This is the time to make the ultimate decision, to fight for your own good, to be selfish, to be able to say "No", and feel free to express your uniqueness.

Now is the time to find out what is it that you really want. What is it that you want from losing weight? Is it to get other people, society, friend's or family's approval? Most likely your answer is "yes", since other people's perception of you is very important to you. But, you are knocking at the wrong door if this is what you believe in.

You have to come to a decision on your own terms. I have written this book to show you how easy it is to meet your goal of loosing weight. I am going to show you step by step how to discover your own road, take your own steps, and adjust it to your own lifestyle.

Step One–Decision

You have to make a decision whenever you are ready to lose the weight *for you*, for your own good, wants, desires and health.

  Step one=*You*=Make a decision for you

List you own thoughts and wishes on staying healthy and fit.

_____

_____

_____

_____

_____

_____

_____

_____

_____

_____

_____

_____

_____

Step Two–Focus

There is this dream inside you that wants to lose the weight and reach your desirable image. Let's take this as our goal, but not as our focus.

Your focus has to stay on you. Your focus has to stay in touch with your soul. Keep your soul in tune with the harmony in your life.

*Step Two=Focus=*Keep the focus on you not the weight.

As we expand all the issues, we will uncover the rules to keep your soul in tune, and find skills to keep your life in harmony and get fit for life.

First, the magic starts in your head, and then you have to adopt it in your heart.

You have to visualize yourself losing the weight.

You have to want it, but just wanting is not enough. You have to want it and love it. Wanting means setting goals and plan of action. Loving means to nurture your wishes and fight the obstacles on the road to achieve your goal.

Step Three–The Fight

Do you really love to get fit and stay healthy? Then fight for this love. Fight to achieve your goal. Fight to win. There are many reasons for having the excess weight.

One reason holding you back from reaching your ideal weight might be that as a child you did not learn the skills of staying fit. Another reason could be the lifestyle you have adopted, or perhaps excess weight is in your genes.

The good news is that now, as an adult, you can get where you want to be. You have the power to decide on what to eat, and how to exercise that is good and healthy for you.

You can change your life by learning the right from wrong. Right eating habits and lifestyle.

You need investigate the resources and skills that will get you to your destination.

We are going to look at the obstacles and fight back to win our lives. Win our lives back to see what is beneficial and what is harmful to us.

We are going to learn the skills and adopt them into our lives for good.

Once you do this, you can sit back and enjoy your life in peace.

Step Three=Fight for your love to stay fit and healthy. Fight to achieve your goal.

Fight to win.

List your obstacles on staying healthy and fit. What is holding you back from reaching your goal?

_____

_____

_____

_____

_____

_____

List you thoughts on how to stay focus on achieving you weight and fitness program.

_____

_____

_____

_____

_____

_____

Step Four–The War

Yes, this is a war. This is a war against all the enemies holding you back from reaching your goal.

I don't want to bombard you with the same philosophies, the same diets, and the same exercises that have not been working for you. I don't want to tell you why they don't work.

I want to tell you precisely what will work.

I promise that when you capture the true meaning of every issue that we discuss, you will not only lose the unwanted weight, but you also will want to preach to those who need it most. You will be their model in their search of reaching excellence for ideal weight and fitness in life.

I deeply feel the hurt inside the people who want to loss the unwanted weight and are not able to do it. I want to fight for them.

But, no one can fight your war except you.

Step Four=Get up and fight for your dream.

Fight for Your Dream

Always remember that life is hard.

Step Five–Skills

When I was in college attending a motivational workshop, Dr. Scott Peck said that the first step to take toward success and achievement in life is to know that life is difficult. In his book, "*The Road Less Traveled*", he says, "Once we truly know that life is difficult-once we truly understand and accept it-then life is no longer difficult. Because once it is accepted, the fact that is difficult no longer matters. When you realize that life is difficult, then you will prepare yourself to win the obstacles.

I want you to know that life is hard, but it is also beautiful. To accept that life is hard, to get prepared, to think like a soldier, to prepare yourself to fight with enemies when needed. The enemies might come to one's life in a different form and matter. Here we refer to enemies as issues involving health and fitness. The enemies like consuming too much sugar and fat in one's diet or not being active enough.

Life might be tough sometimes but you have to learn the skills necessary to reach your goals.

Step Five=Get equipped to find the right skills.

Skills to Achieve Your Dream

What is it that some people successfully come out of problems and some drain themselves?

Step Six–The Belief

These are some of the examples successful people have in common and follow.

- They believe in their dream.
- They stay focused.
- They search to find solutions.
- They find the needed skills.
- They fight back obstacles
- They follow through.

Step Six=Your belief wins the battle

Write down your own thoughts and beliefs:

_____

_____

_____

_____

_____

_____

_____

_____

_____

_____

_____

_____

_____

_____

_____

_____

Step Seven–Winning the Battle

Get prepared to win your battle. Once you recognize the skills you need to reach your goals, you will win the battle.

There are millions of others fighting the same battle like you. Take comfort knowing that you are not alone.

This is your battle, and although you have a lot of support from all different sources.

This battle is yours and you have to lead yourself to victory.

Step Seven=You are the leader.

Write your thoughts on leading your way.

_____

_____

_____

_____

_____

_____

_____

_____

_____

_____

_____

_____

_____

_____

Lead to Victory

Step Eight–Enemies

Step Eight=Recognize the enemies. Find out who, what, and where the enemy is. (we will expand on it later on as we go along).

Step Nine–Allies

Step Nine=Join the allies (we refer to the allies as the forms and matters that are good for your fitness and health).

Recognize the Enemies

Let's look at few examples of our enemies, then later you will be able to recognize these enemies on your own and fight against them.

What is eating you up?

One example might fall into this category. It is not what you eat, but what leads you to eat or not exercise.

Is it a bad childhood experience, peers, family, or career? Are your difficulties too much to handle? Are you out of control to keep your diet and fitness in tune with your lifestyle? Does food comfort you?

In this case, if you think your life difficulties have pilled up and have influence on your ability to stay fit and healthy. Then you have to go deep inside yourself to discover what is really bothering you. You may not realize that it is your childhood experiences, habits, family problems, stress, or not being on the right job that is influencing you to get attracted to consuming too much food, or staying away from fitness.

Write your thoughts on what might be holding you back:

_____

_____

_____

_____

_____

_____

_____

_____

_____

_____

_____

_____

_____

_____

Deal with the real hurt.

Ask for help. Find a confidant that is willing to listen. Find a reputable consultant if you need to talk to a professional therapist. Ask your local church for a counselor. Find a counselor that is right for you. They are ready to help.

Solve the hurt by talking about it, by facing what it is and how is effecting you and the best way to overcome it.

Accept your difficulties as an experience toward a better you.

Accept your reality and let go of the previous hurt. This can be a long process. But, as long as you are in a right track you will get to your destination.

Recognition of enemies is very easy. If something makes you feel down about yourself and shift you from staying on track, then these are your enemies.

When the feeling is unknown or there is a doubt, when you feel sad and out of control, this is when you have to fight the enemy, and fight for your own good.

No More Failure; Be a Survivor; Be a Winner

Get ready to prosper, be happy, and make a positive difference in your life and other people's lives.

You have to be prepared to fight for what you want to achieve.
You have to act like a warrior and a survivor in life.

You have to stand up to the daily life challenges and welcome them as a tool to make you stronger in order to achieve your highest goal in life.

The general rule for winning your life is to be a warrior.
Life is not a box of chocolates. Life is tough. Life is hard. Life is good. Life is pleasant. Life is all.

Life attacks you where you are most vulnerable. As long as you know that life is tough and that you have to fight, life will no longer be tough. The simple reason is that you will be equipped with the best strategy to fight back and to WIN.

Have you seen a leader, or any other successful person, complain about the negative things that have come to them? No, they look at the situation clearly, find a strategy to fight back, and win. They look at the obstacles as opportunities to learn, to get stronger, and to lead better.

The more obstacles you confront the stronger person you will become.

Fight back and live life to the fullest.

Now let's briefly look at some of the major stages that we go through in life.

The main subject is to get rid of any obstacles that have affected your life negatively.

The next stage is to clear any negative past experiences that are holding you back and focus on the life we want to achieve.

Clear the Stage

Here you will find some tips if you have had any problems in these circumstances.

Change your mindset from the hurt toward a positive point of view and look at your problems as learning stages.

1. Childhood

Have you had an unpleasant experience in your childhood that has not been resolved yet?

The first issue to help yourself overcome past problems and not to blame others.

Look into your heartaches from a different angle. Tell yourself, "I have come out of this experience as a stronger person by seeing clearly that those things were not right."

I am going to use my past experiences only to lead my future. I won't allow sadness to take over. I will change the course the course of my life circumstances into a positive gear. Positive thoughts, positive determination, positive imagination, and positive mood toward seeing life.

Negatives thoughts and negative past experiences are history. The positive is my goal, my vision, for now and the future.

I will focus on what I love to do.

I will love myself and will not wait for others to give love to me.

2.   School

The reason for going to school is to learn, to achieve, and to get closer to our dreams.

I will fight for anything that stands in my way of reaching my goals.

I will stay focused.

I will see obstacles as a way of better training.

I will push myself to know more.

I will never stop learning as long as I live.

3.   Love

The aim to achieve the true love. The kind of love that I feel in peace with my life and myself.

I will give my trust to the trustworthy, and I will demand full trust back.

If I fail in a relationship, I won't judge others and I won't assume that all people are the same.

I will take steps to receive the full love I want to receive.

If I don't receive the love I want from others, I will love myself unselfishly to the fullest.

4.   Family

I will look for happiness, harmony, and balance.

If there is a problem in the family, I will resolve it with patience.

I will bring peace and tranquillity to the whole family.

I will respect all, but won't tolerate disrespect.

I will respect all the different individuals with their own unique thoughts and ways.

If my family is unwilling to respond to finding peace and tranquillity, I will stay focused to reach my happiness.

5.   Career

I will achieve the highest in what I have chosen to do.

If I am not truly happy, I will find what I like to do.

Nothing is perfect, but I will enjoy fighting the obstacles, because this is what motivates me.

I am not going to complain about the things that are not there. I will use my brain, power, and resources to find the best way to get the results I want.

6.   Work

At Work I will give my best and demand the best from others.

I respect my team and try to see their qualities.

Everyday is a challenge that I take with love and pride, to solve the problems, to get ahead, and to WIN the competition.

7.   Goal

I will never lose site of my vision. The focus is to learn and learn more. I will choose to be a winner.

I will be a fighter.

I will be resourceful.

I will love, respect, and trust myself.

I will stand up to good values, to protect what is good, and to live my life to the fullest.

I am a winner.

Step Ten–Power

You don't have control over what has happened or what is going to happen to you. But, you can control your response to any circumstances to gain power rather than to give in.

Step Ten=Find the right skills to gain power in any given circumstance.

Skills to Change Your Lifestyle

When I was in college, I was a size six, but I always felt that I was fat. I believe that I was looking for other people's approval, and I was letting society influence me to look like the model on the cover of the magazine.

I didn't look inside to love myself, to be proud of who I am, and to realize the ones who really love me are the ones who truly know and respect me.

I was more focused on pleasing others than pleasing myself. I still work on making the right decisions based on what please me rather than what pleases others.

It is very important to see yourself truly the way you are.

First change your way of thinking to what makes you most happy, then you need to adopt a healthy fit lifestyle for yourself.

Once one of my professors in college said that if you want to lose weight, then change your lifestyle.

If you are wondering how, or where to start, or how to follow through, this is where the challenging part begins.

The Challenge

You have to discover where the problem is.

You have to face the problem.

You have to search for resolution.

You have to turn obstacles into opportunities.

You have to capture your dream.

You have to fight back the enemies.

You need to be true to yourself.

When you realize that life challenges are part of the game, you won't let them take control of you.

Invite Happiness to Your Life

Use your skills to win your life on the road of getting healthy and fit.

Be conscious of decisions you make everyday.

Decisions such as:
- Making healthy choices for your diet.
- Adjusting activities that fit your life.
- Finding your true love and passion in life.
- Being happy with you.
- Wisely choosing the good things.
- Keeping balance with your body, mind, and spirit.

What are considered the "Good Things" in maintaining a healthy lifestyle?

Some people have been fortunate enough to learn how to maintain a healthy lifestyle.

Unfortunately, however, many of us have not learned it. We mainly learn from our family and our immediate environment.

Once on one TV talk show, I saw an overweight woman crying about her excess weight. She couldn't get out of bed, and her family had to help her with daily chores. She was extremely sad that she couldn't play with her kids. The host asked her how she gained so much weight. She honestly replied, "I don't know."

You might have learned and adopted some unhealthy eating and exercise habits that are not beneficial and are very harmful to you without knowing it.

Some people might have learned to eat certain foods that are high in fats and sugars, or some people might consume large portions of food as part of their perceived normal lifestyle.

Not having the skills to maintain a healthy diet and a proper exercise routine can be compounded when excess weight is in your genetic makeup.

How do you change the lifetime of learning the wrong habits?

You do this by doing your research, and by learning and adopting the new skills that are considered "good."

The Skills to Learn the "Goods"

What do you consider "good" as far as your health, diet, and fitness?

We have reviewed some emotional issues that will help you reach your ideal weight and fitness.

The things that are bad emotionally might force you to get comfort from food.

Now let us look at what is bad physically.

- Consuming too much of anything (i.e. overeating) is considered bad.

- Consuming too much sugar, fat, salt, caffeine, fried food, and chips can be detrimental to your good diet and health.

- Consuming too much fast food is bad for your cholesterol and fat levels.

What is considered good physically?

Studies have shown that the following are good for you physical health:

Balanced diet
Keep a balanced diet to promote good health.

Variety
Use a variety of all four-group foods: meat, milk, starch, fruits and vegetables, and more.

Activity
Stay active to keep up with your diet and fitness program.

Adopting healthy eating habits
Change your junk food eating habits to fresh fruits and vegetables.

Drink plenty of water
Drink water or juice with now sugar added instead of soda.

Cook your own meals
Take cooking classes for healthy diets.
Stay away from fast food establishments.

Read food labels
Make a choice of low fat, sugar, or additives.

Research
Read books, magazines, articles, to know more about what is considered "Good" and what is "Bad," for these are going to have a direct influence on your total fitness and balance in all areas of your life.

Avoid Crash Diets

You need to choose a steady method of weight loss to be able to get fit for life.

Stay Active

Stay active; take one step at a time and increase it as you go.

Start with walking at least twenty minutes a day or every other day then make it longer as you get comfortable with the activity.

If twenty minutes is too much at first, make it five minutes throughout the day.

Try to stay active and find anything you like to do, even if it is putting your favorite music on and dancing around the house.

Find an exercise that motivates you. Do you like walking, skiing, running, dancing, or swimming?

You have to be like a child again, think like a child, and capture the fun in the play. Children see life as playtime every chance they get. The thought of play keeps them active. Stay more active with your daily routine by walking faster, parking your car a farther away when going shopping—any little thing make a big difference.

Now that you know some things that are considered good for you, it is now in your hands to control what comes your way. You will be able to make right decisions to select the good eating healthy habits and eliminating the things that are considered bad for your diet and fitness program.

Cherish, nourish, adopt, and accept the good.

Starting your day

Every morning when you get up smile, look in the mirror and say:
"Today is my day,

Nothing can stop me from what I want to be,

I am in control of my life,

I am going to be the best I can be,

I am going to take a good care of myself,

I am going to choose the best for me,

I am eating healthy,

I am staying active,

I can do it."

Today is an opportunity for me to get closer to my dream.

Vision your dream, smile, and be enthusiastic.

Breakfast, Lunch, & Dinner

No food is an enemy if you use it moderately.

You need to learn the habits that support a good healthy lifestyle.

After you learn the habits, you have to read every label, be alert, and protect yourself against the things that are your enemies.

Select foods that are less in fat, sugar, and additives.

Examples of Good and Bad Breakfast Foods

Enemies	Allies
Eggs Whole Milk White Bagel Cream Cheese Yogurt Ham Sausage Bacon Jelly Muffins, Donuts Too much caffeine	Cereal 2% or Skim Milk Wheat Bagel Fat Free Cream Cheese Fat Free Yogurt 4% Cottage Cheese Fruit Juices

Examples of Good and Bad Lunch and Dinner Foods

Enemies	Allies
Too much fatty foods Fried foods Large pasta portions White breads Soda	Salad with fat free dressing Light cold cuts and vegetables Small paste portion and vegetables Dark breads Water and sugar free juices White meat Fish Red meat with less fat in small portions

Dinner

Eat a light dinner early in the evening. It is very important not to eat anything after 8:00 at night; otherwise, all your efforts will go down the drain. The body won't have enough time to burn the calories, and therefor you will gain weight.

Try to find activities that will keep you busy to distract you from getting false attraction to food just for being bored.

Adopt this lifestyle permanently. As you get older, as your metabolism slows, or you get more sensitive to digesting heavy foods, the rule of not eating late at night is another good habit that will keep you on top of staying fit.

Resisting the Urge to Eat Late at Night

Sometimes we have an urge to eat without even being hungry. To combat this, try to find out what is really bothering you. Search for the root of the matter. Is it boredom? Is it the influence of the food commercials on TV? Is it just for relaxing? Is it part of your lifestyle habit? What is causing you to eat, if you are not hungry?

Look into the root of the matter and make sure it is not controlling you. You are in control of your decisions.

Research has shown the urge to munch comes from childhood when parents would give food to their children to comfort them when they cried. You most likely have learned the urge to comfort yourself by consuming food.

Eating Out of Boredom

Do you occasionally eat because of boredom?

Nothing is worse than doing something you don't want to do just because you are bored.

Find activities and hobbies to take you away from boredom. Substitute your boredom with activities to enrich your inner lifestyle. Don't let boredom drive you to eat late at night. If nothing works and you really need to munch, then substitute the munching urges with something light like popcorn, dry cereals, or vegetables.

List activities you can do in times of boredom:

_____

_____

_____

_____

_____

_____

_____

_____

_____

_____

_____

_____

_____

_____

Follow the "Simple Method"

This is a method that bonds with your lifestyle. You will lose the unwanted weight and you will stay in shape all your life.

You have to know that this won't happen over night or in a month. The process of losing weight will take time.

This method is very simple and all you need to do is stay focused on your weight loss and fitness program. You have to:

- Love yourself.
- Value your thoughts.
- Find your passion in life.
- Stay focused.
- See life challenges as treasures in disguise.
- Manage your stress.
- Be resourceful in resolving your problems.
- Adopt healthy and balanced eating.
- Stay active.
- Be consistent.

Let Others Know

It is very important to talk to your friends and family about your mission. This will help you stay on track and will allow others to respect the road you are working on.

Let others know about your desire to lose weight or fitness program. They will respect your way on staying healthy and fit.

My action plan to let others know:

_____

_____

_____

_____

_____

_____

_____

_____

_____

_____

_____

_____

_____

_____

Find A Support System

It is a great advantage if you can find a friend, colleague, or a weight loss society that will help you stay on track.

Find a support system that you can trust in times of need. For example, call a friend in case you get emotionally disturbed by something and have urges to eat. You can also:

- Find a support system to stay active.
- Join a sports club.
- Find a trainer to motivate you.

List your support systems:

_____

_____

_____

_____

_____

_____

_____

_____

_____

_____

_____

_____

_____

_____

_____

_____

Your Best Support System is You

You also can be your own support system.

Find out what is really bothering you inside. Write it down. Find solutions. Deal with it directly instead of finding comfort from food.

List your own thoughts on being your own support system:

_____

_____

_____

_____

_____

_____

_____

_____

_____

_____

_____

_____

_____

_____

_____

Eating Healthy

Choosing healthy foods is highly important to keep you fit for life.

Eat as often as you want, whenever you feel hungry in daytime, but eat a little at a time.

This system of eating a little at a time helps the body digest the food faster and burn more calories.

The energy level stays up at all time.

List your plan of action on eating healthy.

_____

_____

_____

_____

_____

_____

_____

_____

_____

_____

_____

_____

_____

_____

_____

Develop your own style

As you go along and follow through with your fitness goals, you will develop your own style of eating healthily.

Make sure you remember the rule of balanced meals with a variety of foods in your diet, like meats, milks, breads and cereals, and fruits and vegetables.

Never consume too much of anything.
Always keep a food variety in your diet.
Consume foods low in fat, sugar, salt, and additives.
Consume foods low in calories, cholesterol, and saturated fat.
Consume food high in protein, fiber, vitamins, and minerals.
Keep your food intake balanced, varied, and moderate.

Feeling Guilty

There will be times when you indulge yourself and go against your diet and fitness rules.

Some people feel too guilty; they blame themselves for not having the power to control their temptations.

Don't worry about it too much though, this happens to everyone at one point or another.

The only difference between the successful dieter and others is their consistency and persistence.

Write your thoughts on the times you lose track of your diet and fitness program.

_____

_____

_____

_____

_____

_____

_____

_____

_____

_____

_____

_____

_____

_____

Follow Through

You should accept the fact that sometimes you will break the rules.

But don't let that stop you. Go back to your regular schedule and get back on track.

Leave the guilt behind and follow through, even if you need to start from the beginning and concentrate on your dream.

List your plan of action to follow through:

_____

_____

_____

_____

_____

_____

_____

_____

_____

_____

_____

_____

_____

_____

_____

_____

_____

Starting Your Diet

The main reason for this book is to show you how to feel good about yourself, making healthy choices for your own health. And to stay focus on your fitness program.

Every day you have to choose to eat healthy; choose to eat a diet with more fruits and vegetables, and less fat, sugar, and additives.

Consult your doctor to see your chosen diets are safe for your health and fitness program.

List the healthy food choices.

_____

_____

_____

_____

_____

_____

_____

_____

_____

_____

_____

_____

_____

_____

_____

_____

Become an expert

Learn how to shop for and prepare meals featuring complex carbohydrate, fresh vegetables, fruits, fish, poultry, and low-fat meat.

Read nutritional labels and stay away from processed foods loaded with added fat, sugar, and salt.

Become a knowledgeable food shopper and meal planner.

Write down your meal plans:

_____

_____

_____

_____

_____

_____

_____

_____

_____

_____

_____

_____

_____

_____

_____

_____

Crunchy Foods

Some people need to eat crunchy foods.

If you are one of these people, replace the fatty chips with baked ones.

It is also a good idea to have plenty of crunchy, healthy cereals around the house to fulfill your crunch desire.

Popcorn is great for munching, but make sure you use no butter.

List your crunch habits:

_____

_____

_____

_____

_____

_____

_____

_____

_____

_____

_____

_____

_____

_____

_____

_____

_____

Cravings

When poor eating habits pile up, the cravings appear.

The first step to overcoming your cravings is to keep your body's chemicals in balance. You can do this by:

Taking your daily multiple vitamin and mineral supplement. Including an additional 500-1000 milligrams of vitamin C per day.

Take your vitamins with food or with milk if you get an upset stomach. Often, a vitamin on an empty stomach will result in nausea.

Include plenty of vegetables and fresh fruits in your daily diets.

When a craving occurs, deal with it in the best possible way. For example, nothing stops a chocolate craving like eating chocolate. It is okay to eat chocolate. However, you can find a method to stretch the time you are eating it and try to enjoy it more but consume less.

One good method to deal with your cravings is to stretch your cravings. Have a plate of fruits like strawberries, berries, apples, and put chocolate syrup in the middle of the plate and dip the fruits in the chocolate. By doing this, you stretch the time during which you are consuming sugar. Your body gets its cravings satisfied, and eating the fruits will help digest your food better and increase your metabolism.

What are your food cravings? How you plan to overcome it?

Craving:_____

Plan:_____

_____

_____

_____

Craving:_____

Plan:_____

_____

_____

_____

Craving:_____

Plan:_____

_____

_____

_____

Craving:_____

Plan:_____

_____

_____

_____

Avoid Eating by Habit

Do you tend to eat out of your lifestyle habits?

Do you go straight to the refrigerator as soon as you come home from work or school and eat, even if you are not hungry?

Do you eat cookies and milk before going to bed just because you are used to it?

Find your habits and replace them with more desirable ones. Like take a warm bath before going to bed or have a chamomile tea to relax you down.

List your thoughts if you have a track on eating by habit rather than hunger. Add what you can do to replace them with other activities.

_____

_____

_____

_____

_____

_____

_____

_____

_____

_____

_____

_____

_____

Avoid Emotional Triggers

Emotional triggers are another major setbacks influencing your decisions to stay on track with your program.

Avoid trigger eating just because you are happy or unhappy.

Trigger eating like when you are at a party, Thanksgiving dinner, or when you are sad or disappointed at a situation.

Do not eat if you are not hungry or consume less, or eat more fruits and vegetables. For nighttime vegetables are recommended more since they have less sugar in them.

Avoid Situation Triggers

Be aware of the situations that will trigger you to eat if you are not hungry.

Some of these triggers are watching TV and seeing the food commercials or walking through the mall and smelling the foods from the food court.

Stop and Think

Remember to stay focused and in tune with your true body demands of being really hungry or not.

Decide if you are really hungry or if it what you are feeling is a false trigger.

The more you stay focused every time you experience situations like these, the better your decision-making process will become.

Drinks

Drinks are important part of your diet on staying healthy and fit.

Water, water, water. Make water a good friend of yours.

Eliminate soda. They consume too much sugar, chemicals, and additives.

Reduce coffee intake.

Adopt tea and varieties of herbal teas.

Herbal teas also have other advantage to your overall health. Like supporting your liver and kidneys by getting rid of toxins.

What Works & What Doesn't Work with Diet and Exercise.

If you are trying to lose unwanted weight and you have tried everything and nothing seems to be working, then examine this method. Search to see if there is a false trigger toward food and find the real problem. See what is holding you up from staying active and getting in shape.

I like to mention again. Find your dream and your true passion in life. And make sure you make yourself happy.

Choose to make healthy choices, to stay physically active, and to love yourself.

What's Love Got to Do with it?

Love yourself the way you are.

Love your genes, accept your genes as they are, and see the beauty in your genes.

Recognize that we all have different bone structures, figures, and shapes.

Recognize that we have different metabolism, strengths, and weaknesses.

Imagine yourself the way you want to be, in the shape and style you want. Concentrate your thoughts on yourself, the way you want to see yourself, the way it makes you happy and keeps you healthy.

Do not let society, culture, or the size three model on the magazine influence you. Look to the magazines and models for entertainment and do not compare them with yourself. Real life is much prettier. Real life needs your love and attention.

Love yourself, have deep respect for yourself, please yourself first then others, and take control of your own life to stay healthy.

Treat yourself good

Consciousness

Learn to be conscious of what our brain tells you in terms of eating and exercising. It might sound hard if you are not used to it, but as soon as you learn it, it will become naturally yours forever.

Breathing

Breathing well is like filling your body with fuel. The key to energy is filling your cells with oxygen.

Stretch

Stretch your muscles. Move your arms slowly up in the air. Turn your head slowly back and forth. Let your neck and shoulder muscles relax. Stretch and relax your entire body. Stretch is good for relaxing your muscles, it is highly recommended to do before any exercise, helps you breath well, and many more.

Healthy Foods

Add healthy foods and snacks to your diet. Choosing among fruits, vegetables, and dried nuts will not only add energy, but it will strengthen your immune system. Getting into the habit of eating healthy will reduce craving and balance your body weight.

Exercise

Regular exercise is the key to completing your overall fitness. Simple exercises like walking, swimming, practicing yoga, or dancing will contribute to your overall health.

Music

Tune in to your favorite music. Music will help you to enhance your mood. Dance to your favorite music to get exercise and listen to easy music for meditation and relaxation.

Diet

Incorporate a good balance of all nutritional foods in your diet. If you need to cut calories, eliminate chocolate, sugar, high starch foods, foods high in fats, and fried foods. When craving potato chips, substitute that craving with some dry cereal. Don't feel guilty if once in a while you go overboard, just remember to exercise, eat less, and go back on your regular schedule. The rule of a good diet is healthy nutritional balance and sticking–to it throughout your life.

Vitamins

You need to take a multiple vitamin on a daily basis. If necessary, take other vitamins based on your individual needs.

Metabolism

We each have different metabolism levels due to differences in our genes. As we get older, our metabolism slows down. Skip dinner if you have had a heavy lunch, if you feel full, or substitute dinner with a salad, soup, or something light. Eat a little less on each meal. When you don't consume too much then your body has time to burn the calories faster and easier.

Stress Reduction

Manage and balance your life to bring the stress level down. Acknowledge that problems do exist. Seek information to solve your problems.

Stress Management

Life comes with challenges. It is impossible to avoid stress in life. Any given situation like getting married, divorce, moving to a new city, having children, starting a new business, or any unknown situation will bring some level of stress into our lives.

Emotionally, stress comes in life when we don't know what to do with the given situation, we feel helpless, and lack of control. If you open your mind to learn the skills to overcome the situation, then it won't be stressful in your life anymore.

Physically, in time of stress the body releases hormones and increases the insulin levels, which leads to store fat in your body and avoids turning it into energy. This can causes the body to feel fatigued and tired.

In times of stress, your body uses more vitamin C, and if you lose enough vitamin C, your body will give you signals, such as hair loss, bleeding gums, and even depression.

The best way to overcome stress is to learn to handle it effectively.

List the things you get stressed in life.

_____

_____

_____

_____

_____

_____

_____

List the things and places that you can get help in times of stress.

_____

_____

_____

_____

_____

_____

_____

_____

Learn the skills to combat stress

Think positively.
Open your mind to new challenges.

Three Techniques to Ease Stress

1.   Recognition

Recognizing where the stress is coming from. This is a helpful technique to reducing it.

Pinpointing the root of the matter: ""What is keeping me from feeling good today?" "Why don't I feel happy?"

This method of focusing increases your sense of control over the stress. You can then find your way to a better position that makes you fulfilled and satisfied.

2.   Reconstructing stressful situations

When any unpleasant situation happens that you feel the stress, try to write down the things that you can do better, and the things that might have gone worse.

It is important to realize things might have been worse, and more important, that you can think of ways to cope better.

3.   Compensating through self-improvement

When you face a stressful situation that is out of your control, try to let it go. Control your situation by shifting your thoughts to a positive direction.

Take a new challenge to broaden your horizon.

Write your thoughts on how to handle a stressful situation.

_____

_____

_____

_____

_____

_____

_____

_____

_____

_____

_____

_____

_____

_____

_____

_____

Learn to Handle Stress at Work

Everyone has stress in his or her life; however, it's how you handle it that makes all the difference.

We all experience stress over issues and situations relating to our jobs. We may feel pressured to get the work done or we might be worried about losing our jobs. We stew over conflicts and misunderstandings with team members or we might find the work too difficult or not challenging enough.

Besides stress directly related to our jobs, we all come to work with worries and concerns about other aspects of our lives. Difficulties with children, sick parents, tight finances, and lack of free time are common problems for working people.

If we deal with stress poorly, we can pay the price in ill health, accidents, inability to concentrate on our work, and a general feeling of unhappiness.

Here are some tips for handling stress, both at work and off the job:

Decide what you can and can't do something about. You can't do much about the economic climate of the world, but you might be able to help your company survive hard times.

You don't have much time over whether an ill relative will survive, but you might be able to create a meaningful relationship with the person during your remaining time together.

If there is nothing you can do about a problem, learn to let it go.

There is no use getting an ulcer or high blood pressure by worrying about something you can't control.

Speak up.

If something is bothering you, talk about it. If someone else is doing something that disturbs you, let the person know. You don't have to get angry or aggressive-just assert yourself.

Take some quiet time for yourself everyday.

This isn't easy, but it pays off. Use this time to sort out what is and isn't important, and to look for solutions to problems. Even on the busiest of days, it may be possible to get a few minutes alone early in the morning or late at night.

Take some time for fun.

Spending even fifteen minutes a day on a special hobby you enjoy can make it easier to deal with everything else going on in your life.

Take good care of yourself physically.

Get enough sleep and rest. Eat a healthy diet of regular meals. Exercise regularly, at least several times a week. Good health habits are an effective defense against stress.

Take control of your life.

Learn to stay organized and manage your time. Do the most important things first and leave the rest if you have to. Effective time management can get rid of that stressful feeling of being in a hurry all the time.

Learn some relaxation techniques.

Concentrate on deep breathing, using muscle relaxation techniques or visualizing tranquil scenes are all effective ways of shaking off stress and anxiety.

Stress is a normal part of life. Some stress is necessary to provide the incentive to get things done, but excessive stress can be harmful to your health and your work abilities. Learn to manage your problems effectively with the help of stress management techniques.

Fifty Proven Stress Reducers

Stress is a response to a perceived need for action. If you need to do something and aren't able to, the resulting physical and psychological pressure causes stress.

The key, then, to avoiding stress is to learn how to respond to it in a positive way.

Use the following tips to reduce stress. You'll add years to your life and life to your years.

1. Don't rely on your memory. Write down appointments, when to pick up the laundry, when to return library books, etc.

2. Get up fifteen minutes earlier in the morning so you don't start the day feeling frazzled.

3. Prepare for the morning the evening before. Set the breakfast table, make lunches, and lay out your clothes.

4. Schedule a realistic day. Allow time between appointments so you don't have to rush, worry, and apologize for being late.

5. Keep a duplicate car key in your wallet.

6. Practice preventive maintenance on your car, home, teeth, and personal relationships. They'll be less likely to fall apart at the worst possible moment.

7. Keep reading materials with you to enjoy while you wait in lines or for appointments.

8. Procrastination is stressful. Whatever you want to do tomorrow, do it today; whatever you want to do today, do it now! Hard work is simply the accumulation of easy things you didn't do when you should have.

9. Think of your next embarrassing situation as an episode of television's *Candid Camera*.

10. Organize your home and workspace so that everything has its place. You won't have to go through the stress of losing things.

11. Plan ahead. Don't let the gas tank get below one-quarter full.

12. Buy postage stamps and bus tokens before you run out, and keep some parking meter change in the glove compartment.

13. Relax your standards. The world will not end if the house doesn't get cleaned this weekend.

14. An instant cure for most stress: thirty minutes of brisk walking or another aerobic exercise.

15. Take the scissors to your credit cards.

16. Talk it out. Discussing your problems with a trusted friend can help clear your mind of confusion so you can concentrate on problem solving.

17. Make friends with non-worries.

18. Every day, make time for solitude.

19. Resolve to be tender with the young, compassionate with the aged, sympathetic with the striving, and tolerant with the weak and erring-for sometime in life you will have been all of these.

20. Simplify, simplify, and simplify.

21. Say "no thank you" to extra projects you don't have time or energy for.

22. Ask questions, repeat back what you heard the other person say, and repeat back directions. Taking a minute to be sure you understand can save hours.

23. Donate to a worthy cause. Getting rid of what you don't need will make what you do need easier to find.

24. Get enough sleep. If necessary, use an alarm clock to remind you to go to bed.

25. Set up contingency plans-just in case. "If either of us is delayed, we will do this…" ""If we get separated in the mall, here's what we'll do…"

26. When under stress, we tend to breathe in short and shallow breaths. Check your breathing throughout the day, and before, during and after high-pressure situations. Relax your stomach muscles and take several deep, slow breaths. When you're relaxed, both your abdomen and chest expand.

27. Turn "needs" into preferences. Our basic needs are food, water and warmth. Everything else is just preference.

28. Don't put up with things that don't work right. If something is a constant aggravation, get it fixed or replace it.

29. Put your brain in gear before opening your mouth. Before you say anything, ask yourself whether what you are about to say is 1) true, 2) kind, and 3) necessary.

30. Stop worrying. If something concerns you, do something about it. If you can't do anything about it, let go of it.

31. Unplug your phone while you eat dinner or take a bath.

32. For every one thing that goes wrong, there are fifty or one hundred blessings. Count them.

33. Write your thoughts and feelings in a journal to help you clarify things and put them into perspective.

34. The next time someone cuts you off in traffic or stops suddenly, instead of getting mad, think of instances when you've unintentionally (or intentionally) done the same thing. Have you never made a driving mistake?

35. Label situations differently. Are you really "furious" about a certain situation? What if you labeled your feelings "angry" or merely "annoyed" instead? There is a tendency to select descriptive words that are stronger than necessary. If World War II was "terrible," can you describe your flat tire as "terrible"? No, it is just a temporary inconvenience. Putting things into perspective can eliminate or reduce stress.

36. Learn to live one day at a time.

37. Every day, do at least one thing you really enjoy.

38. Be kind to unkind people. (They probably need it the most.)

39. Don't sweat the small stuff.

40. Laugh!

41. Make promises sparingly and keep them faithfully.

42. Remember that the best things in life aren't things.

43. Try this relaxation technique: Inhale deeply through your nose to the count of eight. Then, with lips puckered, exhale very slowly through your mouth to the count of sixteen. Concentrate on the long sighing sound and feel tension dissolve. Repeat this exercise ten times.

44. Add an ounce of **love** to everything you do.
Forget about counting to ten. Count to 100 before saying anything that could make matters worse.

45. Learn to delegate responsibility to capable people.

46. Using the television or radio for background noise or "company" can be stressful. Learn to enjoy solitude and to enjoy thinking.

47. If an unpleasant task faces you, do it early in the day and get it over with.

48. Do one thing at a time.

49. Focus on understanding rather than on being understood, on loving rather than being loved.

50. Train you brain to work on solutions.

Source: 50 Proven Stress Reducers, Stress is a response to a perceived need for action, Illinova University, Decatur, IL 62523

Running on Empty

Make sure you choose a diet that is healthy and right for you.

A good diet will help you stay energized.

Get rid of low-nutrition foods laden with fat and sugar and overcooked. They use your valuable energy to digest and they give you little food energy in return.

When you are tired or busy, it is tempting to live on fast food. It is worth making the effort to replace non-nutritious foods with fruits, vegetables, whole grains, and low-fat protein foods such as beans.

Make water your beverage of choice.
Dehydration can make you tired, so you need to drink plenty of water every day. Try filling a water glass in the morning and continue to sip and refill it throughout the day.

Eat plenty of water rich foods like fresh fruits and vegetables. If your body lacks water rich foods, then your body can become poisoned by its own toxins.

Get moving.
Regular exercise will improve your circulation, which in turn will help keep your body tissue supplied with oxygen. If

your job requires you to sit or stand in one place, use your breaks and free time to stretch and move around.

While resting is important, it is not the only way to fight fatigue.

Instead of slumping in front of the television after work, get up and do something; you may be surprised how quickly you revive.

Substitute junk food with fruits and vegetables for snack.

Get enough sleep.
Most adults need an average of seven or eight hours of uninterrupted sleep to maintain health and to remain alert. Use a fan or air conditioner to keep your sleeping area cool and to mask disturbing sounds from the outdoors.

Practice good mental health.
Look on the positive side of things rather than the negative. Tackle the problems you can do something about: try not to worry about the rest.

Set priorities.
You can't do everything, so concentrate on the most important responsibilities and interests in your life.

List your priorities in life.

_____

_____

_____

_____

_____

_____

_____

_____

_____

_____

_____

_____

_____

Weight Problem

Different genes, different lifestyles

If you have an on-going problem with your diet or ugly fat, then you already know something extremely important. Evidently you know what the experts don't. The problem isn't ignorance about your diet or what to do about the your diet.

The "cure" is one you've heard many times before: "Eat nutritious, lower calorie foods in moderation and exercise (like it or not) regularly.

One answer goes back to your deep down inside feeling that draws you back to food to get comfort.

But, overall you need to feel good about you. You have to make yourself happy.

Another matter is that doctors say you need to look into your genes for weight control. Recognition of your family genes plays an important part.

And the major part of maintaining your desired weight falls on your lifestyle.

The ideal weight for each individual is slightly different from the correct weight. We tend to get influenced by media regarding how you should look and what is desirable and in style. Thinking you are a couple of pounds overweight is different from feeling that you are fifty or more pounds overweight.

However, you need to concentrate on losing the fat if you are at risk for obesity, heart disease, and diabetes.

You also need to maintain a healthy body weight.

Watch out for yo-yo dieting which take you to lose the unwanted weight and gaining it back again.

Choose a lifestyle that consists of regular exercise, a healthy diet, balanced nutrition, fewer fats/sugars/salts/soda, and preservatives in your food.

Love your genes and see the beauty in yourself. Do not compare yourself with the magazine pictures.

Adopt a lifestyle that gives you the flexibility of maintaining a healthy living.

The Final Answer is:

Love your Genes-Love Yourself

Find the cause of your problem

Be more active (find activities that you love to do).

Eat more fruits & vegetables.

Keep it up (consistency is the Key), find a mentor or friend to share your down times, when you feel you can't stay with the system you have chosen.

Find Your True Love and Passion in Life

Life is so real and pleasant when you see the true reality in everything.

Life has more power to it when you find your passion.

Get busy with life and add more activities on to your road.

Make time to help others by doing the following:
Be a volunteer at a local organization
Read stories for children at your local library
Visit a senior citizens home facility
Teach others what you know
Organize an activity-gathering group in your neighborhood

(You can also participate in things like exercise, yoga, crafts, or a book club.
The more love you give, the more you will receive.

Note: The love you give has to come freely and with honesty. It does not mean that you need to please people to love you, or give love back. This is absolutely wrong and will stand against your true inner satisfaction.

When you truly know yourself, and discover the true passion for life and living, then you will give love freely as you go along.

The people who are in tune with you will realize and join the group. The ones that are not in tune need their own time to work on it. If they ask for help, lead them.

If they need time to work it out by themselves, let them work on it.

You work on your own happiness.

Stay focused with your own needs and life's demands.

Be good to yourself.

Lead Your Life

What is your passion? Were you always like this? What is your ultimate goal?

Do you truly understand yourself?

Search your heart and soul.

You don't need to hide behind any walls. Forget about the boundaries of what others might think. You need to keep your focus on you, on what is important for you to achieve in your life.

What is your Mission?

Be clear and stand up to what is important to you, not what is popular or important to others.

Your focus should be on how to lead your life.

You need to take position where you stand, accept life's challenges, fight for what's good, and stand up for your beliefs.

Lead Your Life

Belief in cause: If you don't believe with all your heart and all your soul, then you are not a leader of your life

Integrity: The power is in your personality, courage, intelligence, beliefs, and care.

Noble cause: Stand for something greater than yourself.

Fight back: You will always win when you fight back in life.

Push your limits: If you are not pushing yourself everyday to go forward, then your life will lead you.

Endure pain: You get to know your limits, your abilities, and the power of achievements.

Helping others: In any possible way you can.

Handle pressure: This is the first rule in survival lessons.

Guidance: Stay focused by your words, and your actions, mentors, and resources.

Write your own beliefs on leading life.

_____

_____

_____

_____

_____

_____

_____

_____

_____

_____

_____

_____

_____

_____

_____

_____

Fear

What does fear got to do with weight loss and staying fit for life?

Look inside and see what is really holding you back to achieve your ideal weight and your desire lifestyle.

If it is fear, find it, deal with it, and let it go.

Do you have any fear toward achieving your goal?

Write down your fears so you can find ways to confront them:

_____

_____

_____

_____

_____

_____

_____

_____

_____

_____

_____

_____

_____

_____

_____

Emotional Setbacks

Emotional setbacks might be another negative influence to keep you from reaching your ideal weight and lifestyle.

Emotional resolution is a strong matter that you need to resolve and bring the control back in your life.

Have as many blank journals as you like.

Assign one journal for **you're past memories.**

Assign one journal for **you're present plans.**

Assign one journals for you're **passion and hobbies.**

Assign one journal for **your future desire and activities.**

Write down anything that comes to mind in the related journals.

The past journal

When something strikes you as unpleasant feelings of the past, write it in the past journal and put it away.

Try to find counseling to get rid of the pain and find solutions. If some are out of your control, try to let it go.

Letting the pain go will help you keep in touch with your true self, your dreams for now and the future.

What are your obstacles from past experiences?

_____

_____

_____

_____

_____

_____

_____

_____

_____

_____

_____

_____

_____

_____

_____

_____

_____

_____

The present journal

Keep your rules, regulations, and daily assignments in this journal.

Stay focused with your daily choices. Review it every night before going to bed to know the follow-up for your tomorrow.

Make sure to give yourself credit for all your efforts.

Write down all the good things you have done.

_____

_____

_____

_____

_____

_____

_____

_____

_____

_____

_____

_____

_____

_____

_____

_____

The future journal

Write all your wants, dreams, and desires in this one.

Stay in touch with what you want to be, or where you want to be five to ten years from now.

Cut the pictures you like from magazines and post it in there. This will help you to keep a positive image for you.

Vision and plan a road map for your future in this journal and transfer it in your present journal on time.

Write your vision and plans for the future.

_____

_____

_____

_____

_____

_____

_____

_____

_____

_____

_____

_____

_____

_____

_____

_____

_____

_____

Exercise

Exercise and diet go hand in hand.

You need to stay active and exercise, no matter what.
Exercise doesn't have to be a chore; otherwise you are not going to follow it.

Find something that you really like and stick with it. Any activity that fits your personality and lifestyle is going to work best for you. Consider exercise as fun, a time for yourself, a playtime, and on top of it you will stay in shape.

Start with a little, don't overdue, and expand as you go along.

Adopt at least thirty minutes of an activity in a day.
If this is difficult at first, try to break them into five to ten minutes' activity for a total of thirty to forty-five minutes a day.

Exercise:
Will help your total physical strength.
Increases you're metabolic rate and allow the body to burn calories faster.
Preserves and builds muscle tissue.

Lower body fats and blood fats.

Strengthens your heart and circulation.

Increases your energy level.

Reduces stress.

Improves your sleep, sex drive, and overall appearance.

Slows down the symptoms of aging.

Helps control against disease and ailments.

Find your own routine and:

Stay with it.

Exercise everyday, every other day, or at least four days a week for thirty minutes duration.

Start slowly; increase the intensity gradually over a period of weeks or months.

It is normal to feel tired at first, but stick with it.

Learn the best way of breathing by asking your trainer. Breathe right.

Don't overdo it. A long-term program is the key.

If you feel pain, stop and seek help. Exercise is not supposed to be painful.

Consult your physician to seek the possibilities and what is best for you.

Find Support

As I mentioned briefly, finding support is a great tool to accomplish your goal.

- Find support groups to help you along the way.
- Share your mission to everyone around you.
- Share your goal among friends and family.
- Let them know that you are on a mission. They will help you along the road.
- Find someone to share your moments of uncertainty with, in times when you can't control your urges.
- Talk about your feelings.
- Find the deep cause of your problem.

"There is nothing impossible"

Now you have the magic key in hands. The key to unlock the door.

The magic to hang on to your dream,

And use all your power,

And skills to be what you want to be.

Staying Healthy, Fit and Beautiful for Life

Stay healthy and fit for your own good; it will do you no good to compare yourself with the model on the cover of the magazines.

Recognize your genetic makeup and love yourself the way you are. Pay close attention to what your body tells you.

Balance your diet by eating a little bit of everything. Eat a good balance of fruits, vegetables, bread, meat, and nuts. The key to stay fit is variety.

Avoid consuming too much caffeine, sugar, fat, salt, and preservatives.

Remember to exercise moderately. Walk, run, swim, dance, or do any exercise that is easily adaptable to your lifestyle.

Take care of your brain and soul as well as your body.

Read books, get together with friends, share your good thoughts with them.

Smile, laugh, get massages, light candles, and join cooking clubs, do some gardening, and be positive at all times.

Motivate yourself, get involve with volunteer work, charities, and take motivational courses.

Super busy? Find time to take long baths, relax, and use your chores such as cooking and laundry as a therapy to think and breath.

Learn and adopt the things that agree with you.

Stay motivated to follow your fitness program.

It is hard to stay motivated at all times so have a lifestyle to support you through it.

Set-up environments to promote you to achieve the goals you want to accomplish.

Keep up with a positive visualization. See yourself losing the weight, and believe in your mission with your heart.

Master Your Weight Loss Plan

Now it is time to start and master your weight loss plan.

Is it your wish to lose a few pounds? How many pounds are realistic for you?

Start your plan today by writing the things you need to get prepared.

Keep a journal for writing anything you have captured from this book.

- Write all you have captured from this book in your own version.
- Write down your goals.
- Write how you plan to achieve your goals.
- Write down your mission in your own words.

Plan to go to the library or bookstore.

- Find books on healthy foods (stay away from diet books).
- Find books and magazines for staying in shape.

Keep journals for emotional setbacks

Keep journals for achieving your goals.

- Keep these journals handy.
- Keep journals for past, now, and the future.
- Chart down your needs and plans, as you feel necessary.

Clean up your pantry & refrigerator

- A good search and clean up is needed for a good start. Clean your pantry and refrigerator free of junk foods.
- Start reading the labels on food products.
- Get rid of the foods with high fat, sugar, or additives.
- Buy only healthy foods.

Start with a new monthly wall calendar.

- Use this calendar for your diet & fitness program only. Post it on the wall where you can see it everyday to help you follow your daily program
- Make sure to give yourself credit by staying with your program.

It is okay if once in a while you indulge yourself, as long as you go back to your regular plan.

Stay with your program even in times of celebrations or holidays.

Stay away from unbalanced diets, diet pills, and extreme programs.

Compare yourself with yourself.

Reward yourself by recognizing your efforts.

Normal everyday diet

Choose a balanced diet every day of your life.

Variety–make sure you eat a variety of foods, vegetables, and fruits.

Balanced–ensures consistency and endurance.

Fruits & Vegetables–provide you with needed vitamins and minerals.

Fresh fruit juices–Vitamin rich and an excellent substitute for soda.

No fat or low fat–Stops calories before they get in your system.

No sugar, or low sugar–Ensures your body burns your stored fat rather than sugar.

Plenty of water.

No soda drinks, or less soda drinks–Less calories, less chemicals.

Consume less of any food.

Eat more often, but eat half the portions as you are used to. It is okay to be a little hungry. Your body will adjust after a while and will get used to small portions.

Less white bread, substitute with dark breads.

Variety of beans & nuts.

Choice of good healthy snacks.

Substitute whole milk with skim or low fat milk.

No caffeine, or low caffeine.

Take your daily multiple vitamin & mineral supplements.

Take your additional vitamin C (500-1000 mg) daily.

Never Stop your Research

Keep being resourceful. Find what is good and what is bad for your health.

You will be in great shape as long as you stay on top of eating healthy and staying active.

Best of luck to you.

The Final Word

I want to remind you that this is going to be a long road. Taking this long road is not going to be easy.

There will be times when you will feel hopeless or like a failure. Your old habits and emotional setbacks will pull you down.

You just have to know that these feelings are normal and they show their face when you are most vulnerable. The times when you need help, or can't control yourself, or need to make an important decision, or experiencing a familiar old setback, and the more you will feel the negative feelings.

These feeling will come back and hit hard.

These feelings will pull you down because you are used to them.

Your system is familiar with the experience, and it is easier to give in and fall into its hands rather than to find out what is really bothering us.

You need to stay focused, review your strategies, get in touch with your dream, implement positive visualization, to find out the deep issues that are holding you back, and stay with your plans.

To be successful in your mission is to stay focus, to never quit, and to start all over again if you stopped your program.

This is what you need to do when the feelings of hopelessness come back.

Start all over again.

Search for what is troubling you.

Write your hurt matters in your specific journals.

Go to the heart of the matter.

Search for solutions.

Match the skills.

Make plans.

Motivate yourself.

Join training classes.

Capture your dream life.

Shift your thoughts to the things that you like to do.

Do activities that you like to do.

Call on your support system.

Stay focused.

Follow through.

Take one step at a time.

Push yourself a little at a time.

Resist a little at a time.

Reward yourself.

Constantly love yourself.

Constantly push negative thoughts back.

Just do it.

Just Do it

Just do it might not be an easy answer, but I know you can do it.

I know you can do it because now you know the answers.

The answers might not be enough until you decide to lead your life.

Lead your life fully and remember any little step you take lead to a great achievement.

This road may not be full of roses, birds, sunny days, green grass, and only spring weather.
This is a colorful road with all kind of enemies, wolves, rocks, and stormy days.

The good news is now you know the skills to see the road clearly, to plan ahead, and to overcome any obstacles.
Stay on track and just do it.
Stay on track.
Stay on track.

Stay on track.

Go on. Be the leader of your life.

Recommended Web Sites to Visit

IWeightNoMore.com

This web site is created and maintained by the Author. For the latest information on weight loss, self-motivation and other books and conferences by the author visit this web site.

BzWoman.com

Provides help and guidance in variety of areas. You can also receive personal and confidential help by contacting Jenna (AskJenna) at BzWoman.com.

HowToStayYoung.com

Everything you want to know about living longer. Includes links to the latest developments in this area. Includes guidance on use of vitamins and herbs.

SuccessMotivationalInstitute.com

Need some motivation or enthusiasm, visit the Success Motivational Institute web site to get started.

MillionairesWorkbook.com

This site was created based on the success motivational book "Millionaire's Workbook". The author believes any one can be a millionaire. The book and the site help you find your own way to become rich.

ABOUT THE AUTHOR

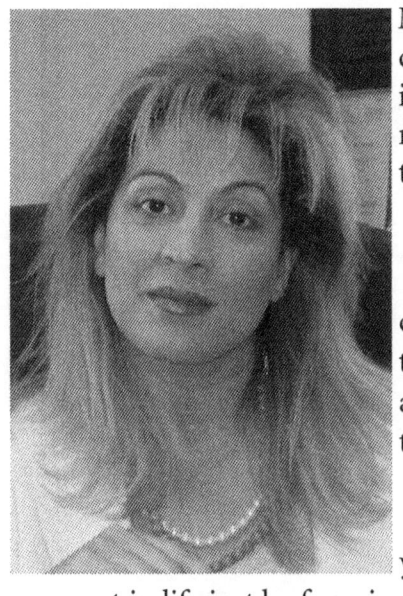

Mera Lord is an author, psychologist, business consultant, image consultant, entrepreneur, producer, writer, director, and motivational speaker.

She has helped people, celebrities, and top executives to overcome their obstacles and roadblocks, and to achieve their dream life.

She strongly believes that you can achieve anything you want in life just by focusing on your desired lifestyle, by being resourceful, and by finding the right skills.

You can find these books written by the author:

Design Your Dream Life

In Search of Answers

Millionaire's Workbook

The Lucky People

BIBLIOGAPHY AND RECOMMENDED BOOKS

1   M. Scott Peck, M.D., The Road Less Traveled, A new psychology of love, traditional values and spiritual growth, by Publisher: Simon & Schuster Trade, Pub. Date: September 1997

2   Mera Lord, No More Failure, Be a Survivor, Be a Winner, Article, bzwoman.com, 2000